INTRODUCTION

Brace yourself as we begin a journey through the story of my life and all the twists and turns that I have encountered along the way. Writing about this causes my emotions to soar intensely, so I hope that I don't get off on a tangent and confuse anyone. My short-term memory is horrible and by the time I am done writing this short story, I will probably have repeated myself over and over and over. This short story could very well become a very long story. Hehe. Oh well, life goes on and on and on and on and I go round and round and round in circles because I can't remember to save my life, just where it is that I was going. I might even be feeling a lil dizzy with every word that you read.

I can still remember when my daughters were younger how we would laugh together every time we would talk about the phrase, "This can't be my life"! With a feeling of sadness, sorrow, and utter disbelief, I feel trapped. Trapped inside a tornado that whirls me in circles; meaninglessly throwing all the good pieces of my life out like they are nothing more than trash. I'm so mad sometimes that I could just scream because, unfortunately "this really is my life". The saddest part of my recovery from brain injury is the fact that I know that I never really recovered as well as I wished I would have. I hate it that I have lost my short-term memory but I sincerely wish that I could just forget that this ever happened to me.

First, I want to say thank you to all my loving friends and family who came to see me after my accident and all the loving and kind souls who gave much needed emotional and financial support. This book is written and edited by me so everything in my book is very original. Every statement or sentence I make is also true to the best of my knowledge and recollection. My only hope is that my book will reach into your heart to help carry you through life, thus giving you the strength to be the person who you truly want to be. You may even have a close friend or family member who could read my book and be inspired not to give up on his or her dreams. It is so important that we all reach out and help everyone that we can. Life is hard and we should all love one another unconditionally. In the eyes of the Lord, we are all brothers and sisters. Sadly, all of my lifelong dreams have been changed now, and I have had no choice but make new ones.

I'm really not sure but I think today is May 18th, 2017. It still seems just like yesterday to me, but it has been 26 years since I suffered a T.B.I. or Traumatic Brain Injury. The wheels of life have rolled me around with no direction or end in sight. Gripping tightly to a dream of a better tomorrow, I have spent more than 20 years struggling without any hope of my memory to improve. I try to stay positive but it gets hard sometimes. Quite often I find myself very upset because I cannot remember what I just forgot! Nevertheless, I'm still very happy that I am even alive today and so very thankful that the Lord has blessed me enough so that I am even able to write this.

Unfortunately, after my accident, I became very sluggish. I would tire very easily and would also fall asleep quite frequently. The impact from the car caused the right side of my brain to be severely bruised. Not only that, but I also had quite a bit of skin torn from my left leg. As a result of the impact, my entire left side became totally paralyzed for quite some time. My equilibrium was also severely damaged, leaving me feeling dizzy quite frequently. Unfortunately, my balance and my ability to walk very well were greatly affected. My short term memory was, and still is, very limited. The paralysis on my entire left side rendered me defenseless and wheelchair bound for several months. I don't know how she did it but my wife would push me around anywhere that I need to go. She doesn't know it but she is definitely my hero! I don't know where I'd be today if it wasn't for her. Being motionless and eating too many sweets ultimately caused me to gain an excessive amount of weight and, I then became a Type II Diabetic.

My recovery has been very slow and continues to be very frustrating. It is almost like I'm living inside myself and being someone I never

Against The Odds

*My Natural Recovery
From
Traumatic Brain Injury and Type II Diabetes*

Vernon Howell Jr. (Pete)

COPYRIGHT 2017

Published By: Pete Howell Publications
Artwork, Photography & Graphics By: Chaz Arthur

Dedication

*This book was very sincerely written to all those who
feel lost and are in need of help, inspiration,
and the proper knowledge of how to be healthy.*

*For my ex-wife Kim for never giving up on me,
my children Kristin Deeann, Morgan Elaine,
Shane Douglas, and my nephews Jimmy and John Howell*

Acknowledgements

*Thanks to the Lord in heaven above,
my family and all my friends.*

wanted to be. T.B.I. has really changed my life forever and every day is very challenging to me due to the fact that almost every time I begin to do something, I will totally forget what I was about to do. Not only that, I sometimes have to drag my left leg along just to get around. It seems I'm always tripping over myself.

Writing this story is extremely difficult for me but I'll pray the Lord will help me so that I can remember everything that I am wanting to say. This book is written by me, yet it's for you the reader. Most of all it is written to glorify the Lord for all He has done in my life. Without the Lord, we all are lost. Since I have given my life to following and worshiping God, I am at peace with every passing day. The Lord promises to take care of us and supply all our needs if we simply obey His commandments. The greatest feeling of all is knowing that all of God's blessings are free to us all. Many years ago, I decided to follow Him, and I've never felt more happy and secure and at peace in my entire life. Never forget, he loves not just me but he loves you as well!

You will probably be on the edge of your seat as you continue reading this but please note that my intentions were never to scare or possibly frighten any of the heartfelt and thoughtful souls who have taken the time to read or purchase my book. Most importantly, I want everyone to know that a portion of the proceeds from this book will be used in the best way I know possible to glorify God and to help those that are less fortunate. Helping the children to become healthy and to be the leaders of tomorrow are two of my main concerns. From the bottom of my heart, I only want to help anyone that I can. My main goal in life now is to change the world for all of our kids, and ultimately make it to Heaven. If I can take this horrible tragedy and use it to help millions of others or just one person then I think all of this was worth it.

Life doesn't always go as we plan it, but we should never lose our faith. I'm also praying that I can either buy or build a place where anyone and everyone can come and share testimonies of what the Lord has done in his or her life. Let us all join to fellowship and bow before God and truly worship Him for all he does for each of us. You will even be welcome to come to dance or exercise or even if you just need a true friend or a shoulder to cry on. I also want to have fundraisers where

Christian bands can visit and perform. We all can sing, dance, and praise the Lord. Wouldn't that be exciting?

The Holy Bible tells us in **Psalm 147:1** *Praise the LORD. How good it is to sing praises to our God, how pleasant and fitting to praise Him!*

As you continue reading this book, you will learn many things about me. You'll learn about my childhood, how I was raised, my teenage experiences, some of my adult life before and after Traumatic Brain Injury, and also my recovery from Type II Diabetes. I honestly feel that my most awesome accomplishment would have to be my three awesome kids! Kristin DeeAnn, Morgan Elaine, and Shane Douglas. "Just Saying".

I do know that I am truly blessed in my life because I can still remember how the Lord came to me long ago. When I was just a child, I used to ride my bike to church all by myself. Now that I am older, I feel that had to have been the most rewarding time of my life. I guess I just always had the Lord drawing me closer to Him. I want you to pray with me as you continue reading this and also want you to feel the chills as I begin to tell you a verse from the Bible that helps me keep my strength and faith each and every day!

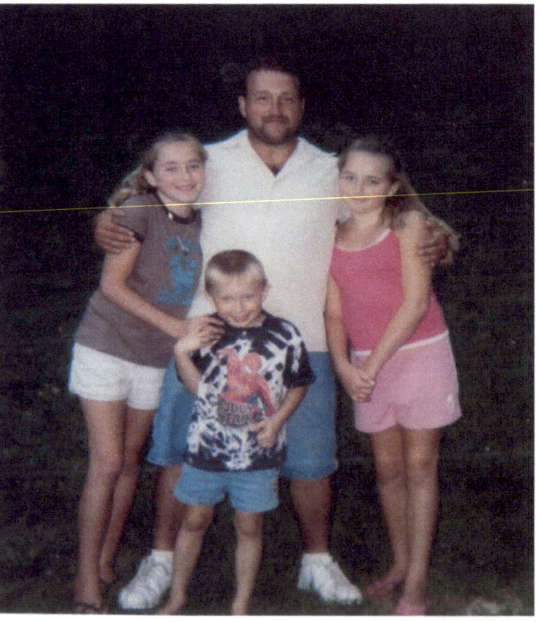

PSALM 23

THE LORD IS MY SHEPHERD;
I SHALL NOTWANT.
HE MAKETH ME TO LIE DOWN
IN GREEN PASTURES:
HE LEADETH ME BESIDE
THE STILL WATERS.
HE RESTORETH MY SOUL:
HE LEADETH ME IN PATHS
OF RIGHTEOUSNESS FOR
HIS NAME'S SAKE.
YEA, THOUGH I WALK THROUGH
THE VALLEY OF THE
SHADOW OF DEATH,
I WILL FEAR NO EVIL:
FOR THOU ART WITH ME;
THY ROD AND THY STAFF
THEY COMFORT ME.
THOU PREPAREST A TABLE
BEFORE ME IN THE
PRESCENCE OF MINE ENEMIES:
THOU ANNOINTEST
MY HEAD WITH OIL;
MY CUP RUNNETH OVER.
SURELY GOODNESS AND MERCY
SHALL FOLLOW ME
ALL THE DAYS OF MY LIFE:
AND I WILL DWELL IN THE
HOUSE OF THE LORD FOREVER.
"AMEN"

From The Holy Bible

I even have the plaque on my wall, "*Footprints In The Sand*". The man asked the Lord where he was at during the hardest times in his life because he only saw one set of footprints. The Lord spoke to him and said, "*It was those times in your life when you needed me most that I carried you*". Give your life to the "Lord" and let Him carry you the way He does me every day.

<u>THE STORY OF MY LIFE</u>

Growing up in a house with three brothers Jim, Kelly, and Dwayne, I can never recall a moment when we were ever bored and had nothing to do. We were always working on something. Dad also had a son and daughter, (Doug and Julie), from a previous marriage. They lived far away but would visit us at different times. Do you remember the TV show, "*Little House on The Prairie*"? I guess we were much like that family in many ways. We 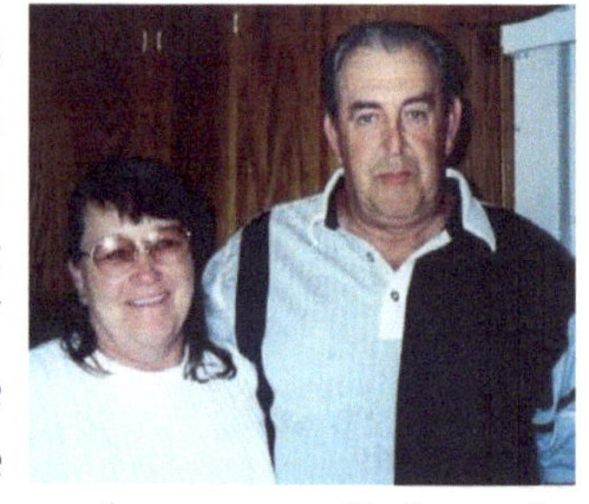 just didn't have a log cabin. We did get our water from a well though. Mom was always outside in summer or winter with that ringer washer trying to keep our clothes clean. I can still see all of our clothes froze to the clothes line in the winter. We really just couldn't afford to have a dryer.

When my brothers and I were young, we would get into everything. We also ate everything we could too. Life was tough, but we learned many values as we grew up. Many of those values have really stuck with me and have, happily, made me who I am. It almost seemed if we weren't cutting the wood we heated with all winter, we would be in the garden all spring planting the food we ate all year. There was a creek right beside the garden. I think every time Dad would turn his back, me, Jim, and Kelly would jump in and get cooled off. That was always so much fun.

I can still remember the day Dad was tilling the garden and all us boys wandered off from our work. We found the neatest arrowhead in the creek. It was so neat looking. It was shaped like a cutting tool and was carved with such precision by some forgotten person long ago. Our land was close to the Shawnee forest so it probably was made by Indians. Gardening can be hard work but those were really some great memories. I can still remember giving it to my 6th grade teacher, Mrs. Mignery, and she kept it in one of her display cases in her room at school. I also remember how Mom would preserve all the food we grew so we always had food to last us during the winter. We grew many different types of vegetables that always tasted so good. Potatoes were always so plentiful so there were always potatoes stored in the potato bin. Me and my brothers had to dig into the bank behind the house and dad built a cellar there. All the boys loved potatoes so I think we had mashed potatoes with every meal. At the end of the season, the left over potatoes that we didn't eat would grow sprouts on them and we would cut them up into pieces and use those sprouts to grow our potatoes the following year. If you ask me, gardening your own food is definitely the greatest and healthiest way to live. The food was always delicious.

I can never remember a time that we ever went hungry. We worked very hard every day just to have food to eat. Besides the food from the garden, we almost always had a cow in the pasture behind the house. Deer meat was always in the freezer too. My Dad was very stern but he was always an excellent provider. When one of us was old enough to drive, he bought us a van, camper, and an acre of land to build a hunting cabin on. Whenever we weren't in the garden or playing sports, I'm sure anyone could find us somewhere in the woods. We all loved to hunt and fish and spend hours in the creek behind the cabin catching anything that we could.

The first buck that I ever killed was a ten point. I was so proud. I don't know how Dad afforded to do it, but he had it mounted for me. Mom was probably mad, but I can still see it today hanging on the wall behind the fireplace. Dad always tried so hard to get us everything we wanted but he just couldn't really afford to. We didn't have very many material things, but we didn't need or desire them anyway. We had love in our family and that's all that mattered.

I can still remember going to my brother's wedding and the bottom of my shoe coming off. It was really hilarious, but at the same time it was a little embarrassing. After that happened, I was a little scared to get married myself, because I was afraid I'd walk down the aisle and the bottom of my shoe could fall off again. That would have been more drama than I think I could have ever handled.

The winters always seemed to be so cold and snowy in Ohio and I hated it. We never had any other heat than wood heat and it was so cold every morning. You could feel cold air coming through every crack in the house. Early in the mornings it just always seemed to be like an ice cube. I really hated chopping wood with an ax or going outside in the freezing cold to bring the wood in, but we had to do it. Using wood is less expensive to heat with but is a lot of work also. Me and my brothers know first hand.

I can also remember the times we would go sledding on a plastic bag or a plastic container in the winter on that big hill behind the house. We would always find some way of playing in the snow. I don't think we were ever too good at making snowmen, but it was always fun trying. Having snowball fights was always great until you got hit in the face. I did learn one very important thing. Whatever you do, don't eat yellow snow! Yuk!!!

In the summertime, we were sort of like the "Flintstones" riding around our go-cart with no brakes. We would use our feet to get it started and then drag our feet to stop it. It was really too fast for us kids to have, but we had a blast on that thing. We had so much fun on it every day until Jim or Kelly crashed it into the creek, and someone ended up in the hospital with stitches in his head. I could have been the one who crashed it, but when you have a brother or sister, you can always blame him or her to get yourself out of trouble. We were typical young boys who were always getting into everything.

I can still remember my brother, Jim, got the end of his finger cut off when the bedroom door was shut on it. I think we all were playing too rough in the house when it happened. Everyone was so frightened, especially Mom. I can still see the big puddle of blood in the middle of her brand new rug. This was the scariest thing ever, but we luckily found the finger and put it in a bag to save it. You know we looked and looked for that finger so Mom could give it to the doctor at the hospital but we never did find it. Now there was not only no one to point the finger at, but there was no finger to do it with either. That happening to Jim was very frightening but there were also many other hilarious things that happened in my childhood. I couldn't begin to tell you all of them.

Life was tough sometimes but Mom and Dad were always the best parents. Dad chose to work as a union laborer all of his life and Mom was an ordinary housewife. However, I do remember that she did have some part time jobs whenever we were younger. It was always such a fulltime job for mom, every day, taking care of us kids. To this day, I still don't know how she did it. I loved my mother and I always helped her cook or clean house or do anything she needed help with. Now when it came to classroom functions, I'm so proud that I was very much like my father. I'm not saying mom was dumb but Dad just had skills that a man needs. He was not only good with scholastics, but he could also fix or build just about anything. Thankfully, my brothers and I learned all of our skills from him. It seemed every weekend that Dad wasn't working as a laborer; the whole family would be together somewhere doing a job on someone's house.

Thank you Mom and Dad for being so good to us kids. My mother is definitely the best mom in the world. She was and still is the greatest cook that has ever lived. I can still see Mom spending hours on the sewing machine using patterns to make the clothes that we wore. They just don't make Moms like ours these days. I'm still very thankful after all these years. I also remember when Dad, Mom, and all of us kids were building the upstairs onto our own house. My brother, Dwayne, was hammering nails right near the edge of the roof and lost his balance. He was falling off the roof but saved himself by sticking the claws of the hammer into my skull so that he didn't fall two stories possibly killing himself. I'm glad I saved his life, but it would have been much less painful to me if he would have just asked me to grab his arm or something. I don't mind at all to offer a helping hand to my brother, but this was a little too extreme. Don't you think? Ouch!

Many of the skills that my brothers and I learned came to us when we did these jobs with Dad. I wouldn't however recommend that you hire us to help you do a roofing job. After this happened I probably would not show up. Roofing is just not for me. My brothers all have very successful careers now and I am very proud of them. This might be hard to believe, but my mom has saved all of the trophies, plaques, papers, or anything we had won while we were in school. Mom was always so proud of us. All of these are probably really dusty but they are all still very proudly displayed on the shelves in her house. She even kept the baseballs from where my brother Jim and I, at different times, had each hit three homeruns in one game.

It has been 30 years since then, but I still feel like it was yesterday. Well anyway, life went by so quickly and before I knew it, Jim and I were in high school. I really enjoyed school so I took all college prep classes. I just loved to learn all that I could in life. My dream was to be smart like Dad and get a good job after I was finished with school. I played baseball for a short time in high school, but I really got into working out with weights and playing football. Playing sports is definitely an excellent way for a kid to develop his or her body and mind. Exercise just seems to give a person a feeling of self-worth.

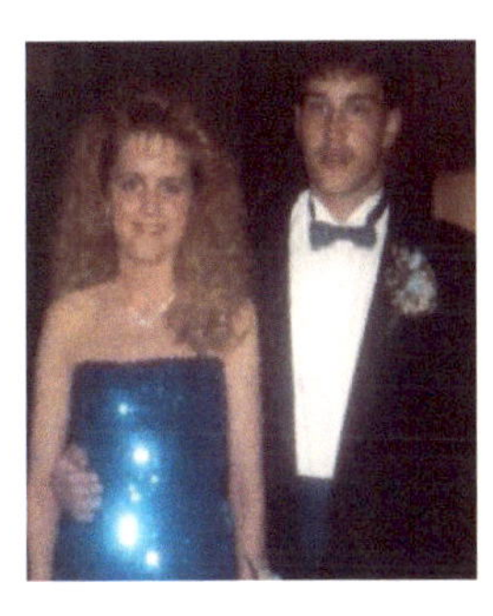

I thought Jim and I had more fun than anyone could ever imagine when we played high school football until I saw his fraternal twin boys playing football. They won

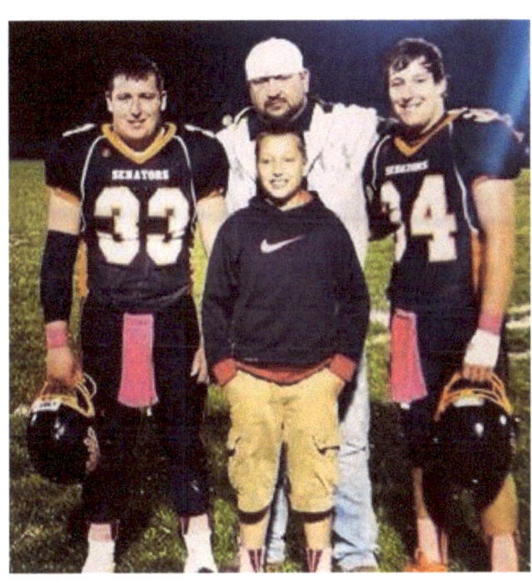

the super bowl when they were younger and they are excellent athletes. They both played the same positions that Jim and I played. They even have the same numbers on their jerseys.

It seemed every time I was going through the line with the football in my hand, Jim would be in front of me knocking people out of the way so I could keep on going. Jim's twins remind me so much of us when we played and it brings a tear to my eye when I'm watching them. Jim and I were always there for each other and I knew that if he was in front of me blocking, no one could get to me.

My brother was a pretty big guy, and he always opened big holes for me to run through. I'm sure if you would have looked up into the stands, you would see Mom and Dad cheering us on. Mom was

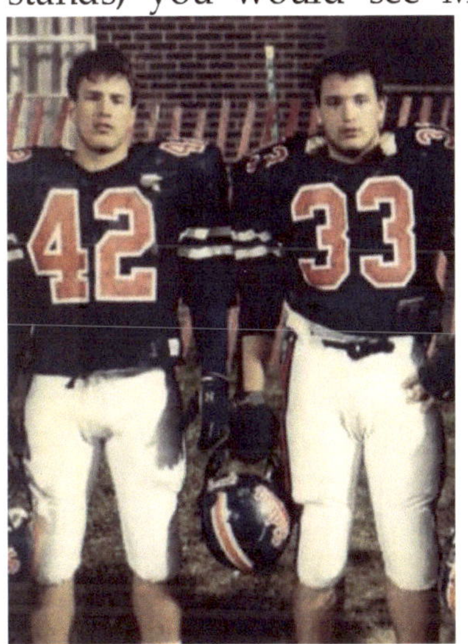

probably crying when she would watch me or my brother running a touchdown or tackling someone. Football is a rough sport and a person has to be tough to play. I don't really like pain and it would really hurt sometimes getting tackled by a defender. I never was injured too badly on the field, but it seemed like a hit of a lifetime when I first saw my high school sweetheart at a school dance. It was love at first sight.

It felt like the 4th of July and my heart was racing. I thought I had found someone to share my life with and I fell so deeply in love. Man was she perdy! I graduated from West high school in June of 1989 and we were married on Christmas Eve of that year. She went to Portsmouth High School and we were rivals but I didn't mind at all. I was young and I thought this was the best Christmas present anyone could ever ask for.   Life as a couple started out great for us. Marriage can definitely be hard sometimes, but we were both so happy.

She went to work at Marting's Department store, and I started college at Shawnee State University in Portsmouth, Ohio. She worked in the candy department so I was always eating chocolate goodies. Hehe. Her Mom and Dad bought us a new car, (Pontiac Lemans), and we were on top of the world. Time just flies and two years in college went by so quickly. I graduated with honors in electro-mechanical engineering technology and I studied all the time. My good friend, Chris Fraley, and I graduated in the same program and soon after graduation we both decided that we would go to Ohio State University to get our bachelor's degree in electrical engineering. This was like a dream come true because I always loved Ohio State University.

My Mom and Dad were very supportive and helped me and my wife buy a used mobile home. It was used but it was so nice and pretty. Well, not long afterwards, we moved it to a mobile home park in Lockbourne, Ohio. Everything was happening so fast, and we all were so busy. We spent hours cleaning and painting our new home, and building a new deck. There was so much to do. Her Mom and stepdad helped us a lot. It seemed like it took a long time, but we finally got it all finished.

My wife then took a job at the Cracker Barrel in Grove City. I was really happy that she went to work there. In my opinion, it is the best restaurant in the country. Besides Texas Roadhouse, Cracker Barrel has some of the most delicious home cooked meals that have ever been made. I ate there frequently and it was so yummy. Over eating too many sweets was also something that I did quite frequently. I really was putting on the pounds and soon began to realize that it was time for a change. Life changed alright, but not the way that I thought it would.

THAT UNFORGETTABLE DAY

My wife now had a job and I was going to work with our neighbor, Mark Rossitter. It was still a little dark at 6 am on October 16, 1991 and Mark and I decided to go jogging before we went to work. Besides eating too many sugary foods, being in college for two years, and eating too much had really caused me to gain a few unwanted inches. I desperately wanted to get back to the person that I was when I first graduated from high school. I kissed my wife goodbye, and she went right back to bed, I'm sure. Everyone knows how women really love to sleep. We lived in a big mobile home park, and it was so beautiful there. It was such a joy every day because there were always deer and squirrels running everywhere.

Mark and I lived right beside each other so we started out jogging side by side. We lived far from a public street so we ran through the mobile home park for a few minutes before we had even reached a nearby street, Ashville Pike. We then left the park and began to jog on the right side of the road. If I remember right, it was still a little dark and somewhat foggy at this time of the morning. I think I told Mark I was going to cross the road and jog in the other lane. I felt much safer being in the other lane facing the traffic so I would be able to see if there were any cars coming towards us instead of from behind us.

OHIO TRAFFIC CRASH REPORT • OH-4 (Rev. 1/82)

LOCAL REPORT NO.		REPORTING AGENCY	N.C.I.C.		
AC-10-91-57	☐ OH-2 ☒ OH-3	Pickaway Co Sheriff	06500	ODHS USE ONLY - DO NOT MARK ABOVE	

REPORT TAKEN	NO. OF VEH PEDESTRIANS INVOLVED	CRASH SEVERITY (CHECK MOST SEVERE)	COMBINED VEH/PROP LOSS	HIT SKIP
☐ AT STATION ☒ AT SCENE	2	☐ FATAL ☒ INJURY ☐ PROPERTY DAMAGE ONLY	☒ OVER $150 ☐ UNDER $150	☐ SOLVED ☐ UNSOLVED

IN COUNTY OF		DATE OF CRASH:	DAY	TIME: MILITARY
Pickaway	IN ☐ CITY ☐ VILLAGE ☒ TWP OF Harrison	M 10 D 16 Y 91	Wednesday	0539

CRASH OCCURRED ON: Ashville Pike
WITHIN THE INTERSECTION OF:

IF NOT IN INTERSECTION: .3 MILES: _____ FEET S OF Airbase Road
(LIST NEAREST INTERSECTING STREET, MILEPOST, HOUSE NO.)

DRIVER-PEDESTRIAN-VEHICLE SECTION

UNIT NO. 1	NO. OF OCCUPANTS 1	OPERATING ☒	PARKED ☐	DRIVERLESS ☐	HIT & RUN ☐	NON-CONTACT ☐	INSURANCE CO. OR AGENT Nationwide Ins.

DRIVER-PEDESTRIAN NAME (LAST, FIRST, MI): [redacted]
ADDRESS (NO., STREET, CITY, STATE, ZIP CODE): [redacted]

PHONE NO.	BIRTH DATE	AGE	SEX	SOCIAL SECURITY NO.	STATE	DRIVER'S LICENSE NO.	OCCUPATION
[redacted]	M 09 D 15 Y 68	23	M	[redacted]	OH	[redacted]	Laborer

OWNER (IF SAME AS DRIVER, WRITE SAME): SAME

VEH YR	MAKE	MODEL	COLOR	STYLE	STATE	LICENSE PLATE NO.	TOWING SERVICE	VEH/PED DIR
91	Pontiac	SUNBIRD	BLU	2DR	OH	[redacted]	Jim's	FROM S TO N

CIRCLE DAMAGE AREAS
Codes: 9 TOP, 10 UNDERCAR, 11 LOAD, 12 TRAILER

DAMAGE SEVERITY	DAMAGE SCALE	VEHICLE DISPOSITION	FIRE
☐ NON-FUNCTIONAL ☒ FUNCTIONAL ☐ DISABLING	☐ NONE ☒ MODERATE ☐ LIGHT ☐ HEAVY	☐ DRIVEN AWAY ☐ REMAINED AT SCENE ☒ TOWED	☒ NO FIRE ☐ FIRE DUE TO CRASH ☐ OTHER FIRE

UNIT NO. 2	NO. OF OCCUPANTS	OPERATING ☐	PARKED ☐	DRIVERLESS ☐	HIT & RUN ☐	NON-CONTACT ☐	INSURANCE CO. OR AGENT

DRIVER/PEDESTRIAN NAME (LAST, FIRST, MI): HOWELL, Vernon J. Jr.
ADDRESS (NO., STREET, CITY, STATE, ZIP CODE): [redacted]

PHONE NO.	BIRTHDATE	AGE	SEX	SOCIAL SECURITY NO.	STATE	DRIVER'S LICENSE NO.	OCCUPATION
[redacted]	M 08 D 25 Y 71	21	M	[redacted]	OH	[redacted]	Laborer

OWNER (IF SAME AS DRIVER, WRITE SAME):

VEH YR	MAKE	MODEL	COLOR	STYLE	STATE	LICENSE PLATE NO.	TOWING SERVICE	VEH/PED DIR
19								FROM TO

CIRCLE DAMAGE AREAS
Codes: 9 TOP, 10 UNDERCAR, 11 LOAD, 12 TRAILER

DAMAGE SEVERITY	DAMAGE SCALE	VEHICLE DISPOSITION	FIRE
☐ NON-FUNCTIONAL ☐ FUNCTIONAL ☐ DISABLING	☐ NONE ☐ MODERATE ☐ LIGHT ☐ HEAVY	☐ DRIVEN AWAY ☐ REMAINED AT SCENE ☐ TOWED	☐ NO FIRE ☐ FIRE DUE TO CRASH ☐ OTHER FIRE

OCCUPANT SECTION

FROM UNIT NO.	NAME (LAST, FIRST, MI) / ADDRESS	BIRTHDATE	AGE	PHONE	SEX	POSITION	INJURIES
		M 10 D Y				A 1 B P C D E F	A 5 B 2 C D E F

POSITION CODES / INJURIES:
1 FATAL, 2 SERIOUS VISIBLE, 3 MINOR VISIBLE, 4 NO VISIBLE INJURY, 5 NOT INJURED

CONDITION:
1 APPARENTLY NORMAL, 2 SICK, 3 FATIGUED, 4 APPARENTLY ASLEEP, 5 PHYSICAL DEFECT, 6 OTHER CONDITION, 7 UNKNOWN

P-PEDESTRIAN

RESTRAINTS

INJURED TAKEN TO	BY
Grant Emergency Room	Lifeflight

RESTRAINTS CODES:
1 NOT USED, 2 NONE AVAILABLE, 3 LAP BELT USED, 4 LAP/SHOULDER BELT USED, 5 SHOULDER BELT USED, 6 CHILD SAFETY SEAT, 7 AIR BAG USED, 8 USE NOT REPORTED

ALCOHOL:
1 NO ALCOHOL DETECTED, 2 HBD ABILITY IMPAIRED, 3 HBD ABILITY NOT IMPAIRED, 4 HBD ABILITY UNKNOWN
TESTED A: ☐ YES ☒ NO TESTED B: ☐ YES ☒ NO

POLICE ACTION

A	OFFENSE CHARGED AND DESCRIPTION	☐ O.R.C. ☐ CITY ORD:
B	OFFENSE CHARGED AND DESCRIPTION	☐ O.R.C. ☐ CITY ORD:

EJECTION:
1 NOT EJECTED, 2 PARTIAL, 3 TOTAL, 4 TRAPPED INSIDE VEHICLE

DRUGS:
1 NO DRUGS DETECTED, 2 USING PRESCRIBED DRUG, 3 USING ILLICIT DRUG
TESTED A: ☐ YES ☒ NO TESTED B: ☐ YES ☒ NO

RECEIVED CALL	DISPATCHED	ARRIVED	CLEARED	OTHER TIME	TOTAL MINUTES
0540	0540	0554	0728		108

DATE REPORT FILED	PHOTOS	OFFICER'S NAME	BADGE NO.	CHECKED BY
M 10 D 16 Y 91	☐ YES ☐ NO	M.D. Evans	32	Sgt. Phillips

LOCAL REPORT NUMBER	REPORTING AGENCY	DATE OF CRASH
AC-10-91-57	Pickaway County S.O.	M 10 D 16 Y 91

IN COUNTY OF	CRASH LOCATION
Pickaway	Ashville Pike at Wayside Market.

General Systems
1005-20

Debris

Kopper's Pole # 7530

A

General Systems
1-1.5AA-14

Measurements

A to H = 33.5'
A to F = 812'
B to F = 32.4
B to H = 78.5'
C to D = 34'
E to E = 47'
E to H = 221'
I to J = 31.8'

A: G.S Pole
B: K. Pole
C: G.S. Pole
D: @ front tire of Unit #1
E: @ rear tire of Unit #1
F: Blood Stain from victim head injury
G: Unit #2 at approx point of impact
H: Debris in roadway
I: Start of Skid
J: end of Skid

OFFICERS SIGNATURE	BADGE NO.
Michael J. Cook	32

Unbelievably, we had actually only been jogging on the highway for maybe a couple hundred feet before this horrible tragedy occurred. To this day, I still can't believe this really happened to me. I honestly don't recall much from that morning so I am not able to give precise details but I am doing my very best. Luckily, I have never had any nightmares. Well anyway, as I jogged across the road to get into the opposite lane, there was a Pontiac Sunbird coming down the highway from behind us at a speed of approximately sixty to sixty five m.p.h. At least from the skid marks on the road that was the calculated speed of the car. The speed limit there was only forty-five m.p.h., so the man was definitely traveling at an excessive speed. Not only was he speeding, but he didn't have his headlights on either. The man was definitely breaking the law, and should have been fined for this.

From what I was told, I don't think he was ever given a ticket. As a matter of fact, I think he tried to sue me for the damages to his car. Well, I crossed the road and the man driving the car evidently wasn't paying attention and didn't see that I had changed lanes. His car hit me from behind and I ended up smashing into the hood and was left embedded in the windshield. I can only imagine the shattered glass and blood everywhere. Mark was truly a life saver, because he kept me alive until the police and ambulance arrived. I'm not sure why, but after the car had hit me the driver obviously drove on for several hundred feet before he even stopped. He was never drug or alcohol tested, so I guess I'll never know if he was even aware of what he had done. I do think my accident blocked me from remembering too much so that I wouldn't live in fear every day.

An hour or more had gone by since I had left the house, and my wife was awakened by someone beating on the door. As her eyes flew open, she was greeted by a police officer. Can you imagine waking up and being told that the man you love was just hit by a car and is being life-flighted to Grant Hospital in Columbus, Ohio? I have tried so hard to feel the heartache she felt at that time. It really breaks my heart and I know I should tell her how sorry I am for getting hurt that morning and ruining all of our hopes and dreams. The life-flight crew that picked me up did a terrific job and thankfully the head trauma unit at Grant

Hospital has the best doctors and nurses in the world. Besides the Lord above, their outstanding work was what kept me alive.

I can only imagine seeing my wife, family, and all my friends standing over me while I was lying there on total life support and unable to live without the use of those machines. I was diagnosed with Traumatic Brain Injury, (TBI), and was only given a ten percent chance to live. The right side of my brain was severely bruised, and as a result the entire left side of my body was paralyzed. My head had begun to swell so large that the doctors had to do emergency surgery and literally drill a hole into my head so the fluid could be released and the swelling would diminish. Reading about a friend or family member getting hurt would always break my heart, but I never dreamed that one day I'd be writing a story about myself and how my own life was almost taken from me.

A couple of weeks went by and I started to have movement again. It was really good news to everyone that I was beginning to come out of the coma.

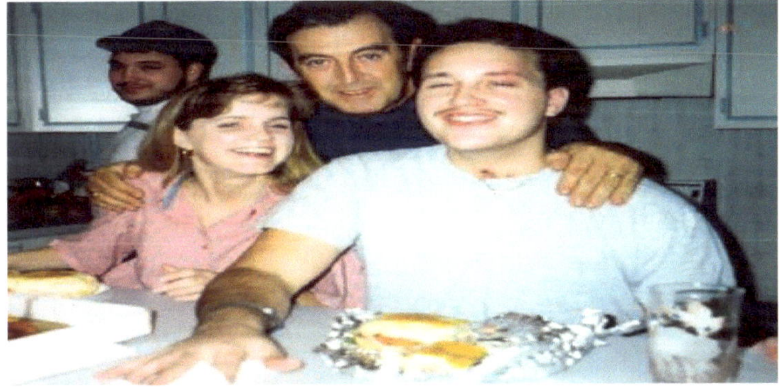

Can you just picture the smile on my wife's face when she saw this happen? I really wish that I was awake so that I could have hugged her.

After four or five weeks, I was released from Grant Hospital and transferred to Dodd Hall, (Ohio State University Hospital). I remained at Dodd Hall as an inpatient from the middle of November until January fifteenth. I know I struggled through therapy, but I was doing fairly well considering the facts. All of the therapist there were amazing and took excellent care of me.

I'M FINALLY GOING HOME

I don't really recall how well I was doing, but I was definitely ready to go home. It was making me so sad every day to see all the people that had been hurt so badly. The floor that I was on was all head injury patients. Some had no arms or legs and they were always screaming and cussing something crazy! It was terrifying at times. My treatment at Dodd Hall was outstanding and thank God I was recovering quickly. I just wanted out of there. Being strapped down to the bed every night and locked in was really starting to make me crazy.

I can still remember that I promised my wife I'd be home for her birthday on January seventeenth so we could be a family again, and nothing was going to stop my dream. Nothing! Besides Mark, the life-flight crew that first picked me up, the doctors at Grant Hospital where I was life-flighted to, all the doctors and staff at Dodd Hall, my will to survive, and our undying love were all what helped me to recover and go home to be with my wife and dog, (Babe).

I don't think anything in the world could have stopped me from getting well enough to go home that day. I'm definitely not a quitter. When we arrived at the house, my wife showed me a big hole in the wall that was between the living room and our bedroom. The morning I had gotten hurt, my dog chewed a hole through the bedroom wall trying to find me. Evidently she sensed something bad happened, and she couldn't get to me to help me. She was the most beautiful and smart Labrador Retriever that I ever knew. I called her "Baby Girl". To this day, I still cry when I think of the love that I feel for that dog. She's gone now, but I'll never forget my Baby Girl. I can still see her jumping through the air to catch the tennis balls that I would throw to her. I miss her so much and I hope to see you in heaven "Baby Girl".

Soon afterwards, I attended about four months of outpatient therapy and it had started becoming even more disheartening to see all the critically injured people at the hospital. Everyday life in therapy was really starting to greatly sadden me, so I decided to finish my recovery at home with my wife by my side. I just wanted to go home! We continued to live in Lockbourne, Ohio for several months, but it really became a big financial and emotional strain on my wife. Driving back and forth to therapy and eating out became really costly. People everywhere were always so good to help us, but everything was so expensive. I want the whole world to know how thankful I really am for all the help that we received.

It wasn't long after therapy was finished that we decided to move our mobile home to Portsmouth, Ohio. Life would be so much easier if we were closer to our families. Her parents were always so helpful.

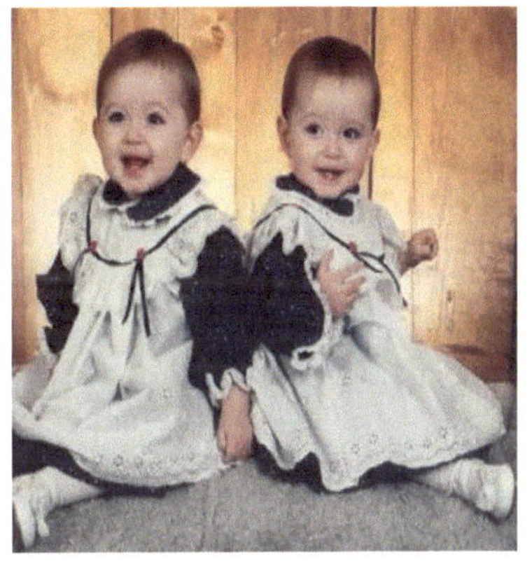

Thankfully, they paid to have our mobile home moved to Portsmouth Ohio. Well, a couple of years after we had moved back, we learned the most amazing news. God had blessed us with identical twin girls, and I would actually be a dad. The girls were born on December fifteenth. They are 22yrs old now. They don't live with me, but I try to teach them good Christian values that will help them to prosper through life and hopefully make it to heaven. In my opinion, they have turned out to be the most precious and intelligent girls that God has ever created.

My accident caused our marriage to literally fall apart, but I have my

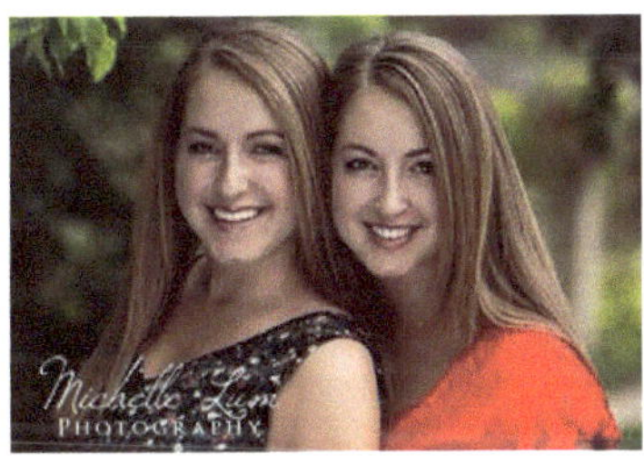

kids now and that's more than anyone could ever ask for. Without my memory, inside I always felt so lost and alone. My wife had to work, take care of our home, raise two kids, and try to take care of a disabled husband. It was really too much for anyone to handle and it tore us apart. I gave my wife our home so that my girls would have a good place to live and I moved in with my Mom and Dad. Soon afterwards, my Dad bought me a mobile home and put it on the land above their house.

It was at this time in my life that my son was conceived. Unfortunately, his mother and I are no longer together either. I have the worst luck with relationships. I'm so happy though that my son is a very good athlete. He is 17 years old now and might even be the next new "Pete Rose". It makes me so happy when I watch him play baseball. He is very talented and I think he is going to follow in his Dad's footsteps. I was at one of his games last summer, and all I could do was cry.

Anyway, I truly loved living above my parents. I was safe there and knew I always had a home of my own. It was so beautiful, but after living there for several years I started to get very annoyed by the woodpeckers and the fact that you couldn't get up the hill to my house in the winter, because it was very steep.

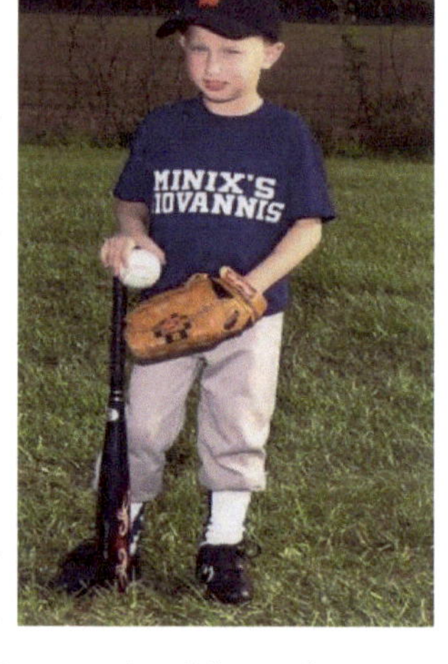

I decided to move to town so I could be closer to my friends and have more activities to do. After my accident, I had so much free time. I should have been exercising but all I did was sit around and eat. I gained a tremendous amount of body fat and developed Type II Diabetes. My memory and balance were definitely so bad that I wasn't able to keep a job. I really shouldn't have lived alone but at least my parents were close by. To pass the time, I would visit different nightclubs at least three or four nights a week.

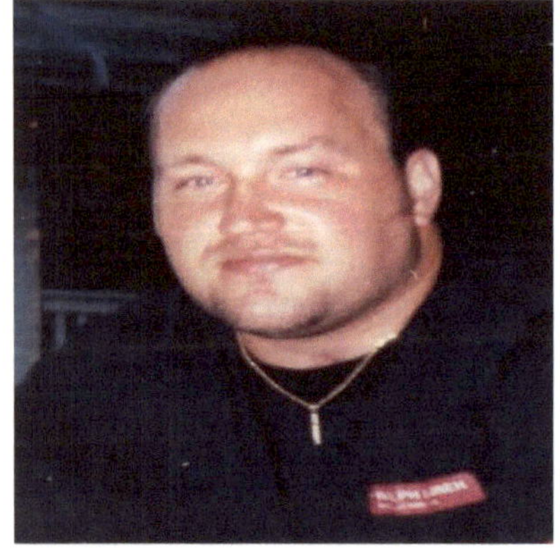

Dancing has always been so much fun to me and I was still fairly good at it even after my accident. At least I thought I was. As a matter of fact, I think Michael Jackson was my hero when I was a teenager. That man could really dance.

My Mom still has the trophy that I won first place in a dance contest in maybe the sixth grade. Dancing and school were and still are my two big passions. When life gets hard, just turn on the music and dance or exercise.

YOU OUGHT TO SEE ME NOW!

One summer night I was dancing at a nightclub, and I met a gentleman whom became my landlord, life coach, and my personal trainer. After living in the apartment above him for some time, I began to realize what a genius he really was. He showed me how to lose the forty-five to fifty pounds of unwanted fat, and how to keep it off with exercise and all natural fitness drinks that he taught me how to make. These all natural, very inexpensive fitness drinks were actually made of organic apple cider vinegar mixed with other juices. I started feeling great and full of energy. I was finally getting back to the person that I used to be.

By eating healthy, exercising frequently, drinking these drinks, "eating Mega Greens" that I purchase from Lyon Legacy, and my using my, "Ab Coaster" that I purchased from an infomercial, I can honestly say that I no longer have any symptoms of Type II Diabetes. Amazingly, I lost five inches from my waistline. Through my research, I have learned that apple cider vinegar is actually very effective for many different things. In regards to my healing, the medications that I took while I was in the hospital were very effective in relieving the pain that I was experiencing. However, I learned that your body actually has its own healing energy called your "Chi". For so many years I felt so tired and in pain and discomfort until I learned all about how to become healthy, naturally.

People overdose on medication every day. "Just saying". Have you ever heard of anyone dying from an overdose of nutrition? Never! You probably haven't. Therefore, I have come to the conclusion that medication may kill and nutrition may heal. We should do our very best to stay healthy. A very wise man named Hippocrates once said, "*Let food be your medicine and medicine be your food*".

Corinthians 6:19 in the bible tells us *What? know ye not that your body is the temple of the Holy Ghost [which is] in you, which ye have of God, and ye are not your own?*

The Lord has blessed me tremendously and I'm very thankful to be the person that I am today. I'm not a licensed personal trainer but I have acquired the knowledge that can hopefully help to make any person's body to become healthy and pain free. I had pains in my shoulder that were unbearable for many years after I was injured. Cortisone shots were injected into my shoulder two different times. These shots were effective for a couple of months, but the pain would eventually return. It became totally unbearable. My shoulder would hurt so bad that I couldn't even handle the pain from wearing a heavy coat in the winter. I used a small, all natural, inexpensive, and pain free device called a "Stimulator" to fix this problem.

Amazingly, this mechanical device shoots small electrical signals through your body and repairs damaged tissue. My shoulder had hurt for years and unbelievably in a few seconds that device totally cured me of a life-time of pain. I am still completely amazed at how my shoulder has been healed after all those years of pain and discomfort. I am not sure but I think I still may even be able to purchase these for anyone who may want to try it.

The other product that he ordered for me from Lyon Legacy was a "magnetic skull cap". This is the product that allowed me to be able to sleep in my bed again and actually get a full night of sleep. For so many years I had to sleep in a chair. Getting in and out of the bed would make me very dizzy. This cap also helps me to think much more clearly every day. Seeing and feeling the progress that I have made by using this cap makes me so happy. Before I purchased this product, I could hardly even bend over without losing my balance. There was no way I could ever lie flat on my back without my head spinning very fast. It spun so fast that I would feel like I was going to vomit.

The magnetic skull cap is truly a godsend. This magnetic skull cap is also

effective in relieving migraines, restlessness, tumors, or any head or brain related injury. Amazingly, I am pain free, full of life and energy now and able to do the things I want and need to do each day. That is if I can remember what I need to do.

On my website, **www.getfittoenjoylife.com,** you will see a testimonial from a girl who had Multiple Sclerosis. I recommended to her that she try the magnetic skull cap. She purchased one and wears it to bed every night. It is unbelievable the healing that she experienced. I think besides wearing the skull cap, I also recommended that she also detox her body with herbs. As of today, she no longer has seizures or requires any of the seizure medication that she had taken for so many years.

I have personally seen and experienced the true healing power of magnets. Magnetic and nutritional products from Lyon Legacy are what I recommend to anyone who is trying to heal his or her own body. Go to the website, **www.lyonlegacy.com,** and read all about why and how magnets heal your body. I'm so happy for my healing and I love to be able to help others. Besides organic apple cider vinegar, Lyon Legacy's products have helped to heal my body in ways that I never dreamed were possible. I can't thank them enough for everything they have done for me.

Natural healing is possible without the use of any pharmaceutical drugs. Keep in mind that I also have access to a silver substance called "colloidal silver" that will kill all one celled pathogens, parasites, or viruses. I personally haven't been sick for twenty years or more. My allergy problems are even gone now. All I did was use a glass eye dropper and squirt this down my nasal passages. Also, I no longer get fever blisters after I applied this to my lip. This is definitely a truly amazing product. It is also great to help heal poison ivy and removing acne.

After being healed myself, I now have the knowledge on naturopathic healing and nutrition that may help anyone to recover from an injury or to help maintain his or her health. Educate yourself, don't medicate yourself. From childhood through adulthood we learn that we need vitamins and nutrition to keep us healthy. Is there any need for medication? The Bible says God gave us every herb of the earth to keep us healthy. I highly recommend that you use the Bible as a guideline for your life.

> **Genesis 1:29** *And God said, Behold, I have given you every herb bearing seed, which [is] upon the face of all the earth, and every tree, in the which [is] the fruit of a tree yielding seed; to you it shall be for meat.*

The story of my life is proof of everything I have told you, because I have the pictures and the documents to prove it. You can reach me on the web at: **petehowell1971@outlook.com** or **www.getfittoenjoylife.com**, and see the changes that I have made in my life and appearance.

Being happy and healthy are possible with the use of these all natural products. You can find all of these I've mentioned and other biblical recommendations in my other book," **Healthy Healing Talks**".

God bless everyone and please remember to pray and live your life for the Lord. I hope my book has touched you the way it did me when I first wrote it for you!

This was the story of my life. I not only learned it... I lived it.

By: Vernon Howell Jr. (Pete)

God bless everyone and thank you for reading my book.
Vernon Howell, Jr. (Pete)

Call ...
(740) 935-7905
anytime to order products or set up a
Healthy Healing God-filled presentation or an inspirational
and informative exercise party.

You Can Make Real, Definite, Positive Changes To Your Body
When You Start A Regular Healthy Routine.
Come On, You Can Do It Too!

BE AWARE . . . BE HEATHY . . .
AND
"GET FIT TO ENJOY LIFE"

I will come and speak to you or your:
• Church • Youth Group • Study Group
• School Group • Sports Team • Club
• Small, In Home Group...

Please call for more information or to set up a date and location for your presentation or healthy healing inspirational/motivational consultation. Prices are reasonable and negotiable and are for travel costs, hand-out materials and to help me continue to inspire others. I will share with you how God's healing blessings have helped me to recover my health more each day and can help you to become healed also.

Books will be available at seminars
for $19.95 or 2 for $30.00

www.getfittoenjoylife.com
or Email:
petehowell1971@outlook.com